CANCER: WE BEAT YOU

FOREWORD

So I want to start off by saying that this isn't a morbid tale, or me looking for sympathy. This is me writing about my feelings and the challenges I faced when my mum had cancer.

Cancer is a scary word and even scarier when you're a teenager trying to cope with the fact his mum has cancer. I liked to bottle things up and it wasn't good for me.

I'm writing this for two reasons, one because this is a story that needs sharing, as no one understands how it feels when you mum has cancer and you have to continue with your life like nothing has happened. Secondly I want this to help people who may be going through a similar situation or help people supporting someone in this situation understand better what they might be going through.

After all this isn't a situation there is a self-help book for. It isn't a situation that happens every day and you never expect to be in the situation. It would've really helped me to read what someone else had been through and how they'd felt, it would've helped me to make sense of my feelings and realise that they weren't wrong.

So here's my story

PART 1 – DIAGNOSIS AND EARLY DAYS

So this starts off about me as the first memories I have are of me being really busy at school. I had to prepare a presentation for my English GCSE. The mark of this presentation went towards my GCSE English exam, and I really wasn't prepared for it. Others had gone before me with these spectacular presentations full of experiences and everyone came across really confidently. My life just wasn't like that, I didn't have anything to share and I certainly wasn't going to come across confidently at all. It also needed to be good as I wanted to impress a girl in my class (who doesn't in high school?).

The story starts like this because it shows that I wasn't different, I was a normal teenage boy at this time, stressed about GCSEs and trying to impress a girl. Life didn't really change that much school-wise and this was important for me, as you'll see.

The first thing I noticed was that my mum was home a lot more. She used to be really busy getting ready for work in the mornings and now some mornings' she wasn't and she would spend a lot more time with us before we went to school. I didn't really think a lot of this as my mum has always been there for me both after and before school. My dad however works long hours and so when he started being home with my mum some mornings I did start to think something was going on. I know this sounds odd but I suppose it's the little things that you pick up on first and I didn't really think much od all of this at the time, just that it was odd. It actually annoyed me a little at the time as I like having time alone and suddenly there wasn't this time anymore as my mum (understandably) wanted to spend more time together and this was hard for me. This sounds selfish but I needed that time for me and it really messed me up, including my mood.

***

One afternoon after I had finished school it was just my mum and I in the house, I could see that my mum was upset and I wanted to know what was up. Now my mum isn't usually someone who cries at all, she's a really strong person so I knew it was something really big. She then told me all about the appointments and referral to the hospital, I knew why she had been home many times and also I started to get worried. Soon we were both hugging and crying at the bottom of the stairs. All I remember from that moment was staring at the white banister. I didn't cry for long, I was more in shock. I didn't know what to say. I didn't know what to do. At that moment I felt kind of hollow, the diagnosis wasn't yet confirmed but yet both my mum and I knew what the test results would say. She wanted to prepare me.

I remember that I just felt isolated. This feeling hasn't ever really gone from that day. I suddenly became different. I suddenly became someone who no one quite knew how to approach.

***

The next day I was expected to carry on completely normally. What else could I do? I went into school and remember that it wasn't too bed. Definitely wasn't as bad as I was expecting. I had already told my closest friends over text message and this did make my whole day easier as they already knew. I didn't have to tell them face-to-face. I don't know how I would've managed that. Many of my friends were really great, they were there for me through it all and made things as normal as they could at school. This normality and joking around as normal was just exactly what I needed. School was an escape for me and increasingly this became the case. I did however have friends that acted weird around me after they knew and you can't blame them. What are you supposed to say? I always thought that it was as difficult for them as it was for me.

I thought I was doing really well as it approached lunchtime on that first day. I had survived the morning and I was feeling quite good. I then realised that I needed to tell my English teacher. Face-to-face. This was because I was supposed to be doing my presentation today. I froze. I started to panic but my friends stepped in and supported me. I told my English teacher, I can't remember what I said but I held it together and that's all I wanted to be able to do. This was hard because it made me accept what was happening.

Nothing was a shock after everything that had happened, so when the diagnosis was confirmed that evening, nothing felt different. My mum had cancer.

***

The days after this everything blurred into one. Things happened so fast after that. It was good as my mum was getting the treatment she needed but it gave me no time to keep up with everything or make sense of what was happening. I felt like I needed to reach out to someone but I couldn't. What could I say? What difference would they make?

I did reach out though. I talked a lot to my grandma. I told her how I felt distant from everything that was happening, like it was happening to another family and I was simply observing. I also asked her why a lot. I just couldn't accept what was happening.

Not a lot happened after all the initial shock. My mum had a review with two different consultants who presented her with two different options for the surgery. We didn't know the prognosis yet but it had been caught early. My mum not recovering didn't even enter my head

PART 2 – SURGERY AND CHEMOTHERAPY

The day my mum went in for her surgery was pretty much the same as any other day; I went to school and remember being really worried all morning. I couldn't concentrate. By this time all my teachers knew and they kept asking me how I was. This isn't what you want to be asked when you don't know truly how you feel, but it was nice to know they were there for me. It became a reflex just to say "fine" or another noncommittal phrase.

The morning really dragged on and I just wanted to know hat had happened, I didn't think I could've been there waiting. Just sitting in school not knowing was enough, I was aching to find out. At lunchtime the wait was over, everything had gone really well and they had removed the tumor. Good news.

I went to see her in hospital that evening with the rest of my family. She seemed so bright that I still couldn't and therefore didn't believe she was ill. She was bright and smiling and didn't look ill. These facts allowed me to remain detached. Allowed me to keep with this coping mechanism I had built up. The reality of the situation did hit me that night though, I realised that there was a long road ahead.

The next few weeks past by without anything really happening. Mum was home again and things kind of went back to normal. At this time we all regained a positive vibe and time in the house was nice. We got the biopsy results and even though the news was worse tan expected everyone stayed positive. It was still treatable. Chemotherapy and Radiotherapy.

This didn't worry me at the time, I was just glad she was home. I also didn't understand the effects the Chemo would have on my mum. I'd never seen it before so why should I? I think my mum told me about the side effects but I'd taken tablets before and they had a whole bunch of side effects that I didn't get so I just presumed it was like that. My mum wouldn't get any of them, surely? I remember having conversations with my mum about hair falling out and sickness and also what happened at the chemo appointments. I still think it wasn't real for me and even though the conversations were supposed to prepare me for what was going to happen, I never think you can be fully prepared.

The first Chemo sessions passed and not a lot really happened, there wasn't a lot of difference initially as things take time to happen. However every night after each Chemo session was terrible, even though mum was on anti-sickness meds she was still violently sick. It was only the night but it was after each Chemo session. It often kept me awake and it obviously wasn't nice to listen to. It really made me again question why this was happening to us. The next morning, without fail she was always fine. Well the sickness was fine. She was tired and had other symptoms at this point.

I also realised how much my mum did for us all, selfishly I noticed this when I had to do more to help around the house. This was really hard to accept at first and our lives became more hectic. I had to grow up very quickly and this was hard.

I actually learnt a lot about myself during this time and it taught me how strong I could be and I loved the feeling of being an emotionally strong person. I wanted to keep that up, no matter what the cost. It also taught me how adaptable to change I am and how this could be good for the future.

Soon after these first few sessions they became harder on my mum. Fevers and infections were common, no matter how careful we all were with hygiene in the house. The infections could be really serious and life-threatening unless she got treatment which sounds like a flippant comment, like I'm exaggerating, but it's true. Chemo makes it the truth unfortunately. She often had to be rushed into hospital late at night. The first time this happened I was scared, really scared. I didn't know what was going to happen and all the next day at school it was impossible to concentrate. It just felt like I was on autopilot the whole entire day and the other days when this happened. It got more frequent towards the end of the Chemo and therefore more scary.

I knew that my mum would want me to stay in school and continue with my exams so that's what I did. I kept visiting her in hospital though and the number of times I did that over this period was large. I can't remember the number. Just that each time I just presumed she would get better each time and luckily she did. I don't know what I would've done if she didn't get better, I just never even considered it. After the first few times it wasn't scary any more. I even had to take my GCSE revision into the hospital so I could revise with my mum. It was a difficult time and one that really tested me. It was difficult to get my revision done but it was also difficult to actually spend any time with my mum. I felt like at this time I hardly saw her.

However it all worked out, my mum finished all her chemo sessions without any major incidents and I think the hardest thing by far was my mum losing her hair. This was hard for her and me because the wigs were nice but nothing like her natural hair. I never realised what a big change this was until it happened and it took a lot of getting used to, there were the wigs and then sometimes she wore a scarf on her head instead and I'm still not sure how I felt about that. It was just weird. It was a constant reminder she was ill. Other things in my life were either normal or I could pretend they were normal but not this. It was a visual reminder and one that was around constantly.

PART 3 – THE CAREER CHOICE AND FURTHER TREATMENT

Seems like an odd title? Well this whole experience so far has been quite bleak and shows how devastating Cancer can be to the whole family however I had have a major positive come out of it. It made me realise what I wanted to do with my life.

I'd visited my mum a lot in hospital and this made me realise that I wanted to work in healthcare. It sounds cheesy but the whole experience of seeing how good the doctors and other healthcare professionals were to her and how much compassion and knowledge they had. This further set my mind at ease that when she was in hospital she was looked after well. All the qualities these people showed I wanted to develop and that really sparked my interest in a career path I'd never thought about before. It was a goal and I know it made my mum happy to know that I was thinking about the future and she could start planning how we were going to get there together.

Things also progressed to the future for my mum as she had finally finished all her chemotherapy. I was also glad I didn't have to come to the hospital to visit her again, and worry what I might find. I will never see that hospital in the same way again, all those evenings standing in the car park waiting for my dad to lock the car so we could go inside. Not wanting to go in but pushing myself. It was all over. It was a really happy time when she came home following her final treatment session and we were all so relieved she had made it through her chemotherapy. During this time she also went to a support group that had been set up by fellow patients at the hospital.

This support group was so good for my mum as I think the fact that others had beaten it made her realise that she could do it too and that there was a future. They did meetings where they could all talk and kind of social gatherings too. My mum always came back full of positivity and even though she never really connected with the meetings and stopped going once she recovered, I think she didn't really understand the effect the positivity had on us as a family. The way she talked about the people there really gave me hope of a return to the norm after the cancer had been dealt with.

***

Radiotherapy was nowhere near as bad as the chemo in terms of the side effects my mum experienced. Nothing really changed and slowly but surely we started to return to normality. Mum was still off work and attending her radiotherapy sessions but she was a lot less 'ill'. We started to talk a lot more at this stage and she started to open up about her treatment and how she felt. However I still felt like I couldn't ask questions as I didn't want to upset her so these conversations were still quite one-sided. I just couldn't know what my mum was going through when I was a school, I just didn't think I could handle it all in one go like that. Now the worst was over though I wanted to know more than ever.

I was sitting on the corner of the bed and she told me everything. How the chemo had effected her and how the radiotherapy worked and it all had a really strange effect on me, I regretted not being there through all the treatment. I wished I'd been at the treatment session, it made me really sad. I knew this couldn't be helped as I had school but I still wished I had been there.

Speaking to mum also made me realise how she got through it all. She had a mental checklist of sessions and after each session she ticked it off. This gave her such determination and strength and I really admired that. Now there weren't any sessions left. My mum had beaten cancer. Our lives could go on.

PART 4 – RIGHT UP UNTIL THE HERE AND NOW

The day the all clear came it was amazing. The correct term is remission as they never like to say that you're cured as the cancer can come back. This didn't stop our happiness however and we celebrated with champagne and had all the family over. It was a really nice day and we really celebrated what we had all been through together. Already at this time I couldn't properly feel happy, I didn't think anything of it though as I had my GCSE results coming up. I've struggled to have any proper feeling since.

After this party life continued. Mum's hair grew back and I had good news too – I got into sixth form with my GCSE grades.

In sixth form everything was normal, mum went back to work and still went for some appointments to check that everything was still okay, but to this day there's never been a scare that the cancer is coming back.

Things changed for me though, I started to struggle. Up until this point I'd never struggled at school, I'd always got what I wanted but suddenly there was pressure. I had a plan and that plan needed me to get good grades in my A-Levels. As things got tough I started to panic mire and more but I kept all this to myself. My family were happy, why should I worry them?

My family did start to notice though and just put it down to exam stress. I mean it's only natural. I never linked any of the problems I was having my mum's cancer. I just never thought that after everything had gone fine I would still be affected by it. Even when I got into University to study Physiotherapy like I wanted to do I didn't feel 'right' I felt happy, don't get me wrong, but I didn't feel as happy as my friends and I didn't even feel like it was happening. It was like I was in a daze constantly. Numb to what I was feeling.

Therefore I went to University without having properly dealt with my feelings. The first few weeks in that new environment were terrible. I missed home so much and cried. I haven't even properly cried when my mum was ill. However after those first few weeks I managed to get through my first year without any major problems. I had a great time in fact, and the year passed by like a blur. I never thought any more about my feelings but more and more I struggled to drag myself from my bed. Some days I just couldn't do what I wanted to do, but at this time I had so many good days where I had such a good time that I didn't think about it.

I only started to think about all of this further during my second year at University. It all started with me joining the mixed Hockey Team. I'd loved playing Hockey (field hockey) since school and decided that this year I would make myself join the team and meet some people who were outside of my course. I loved it. Initially I went to every training session and every social. It was a great time and I met so many great people. I was so happy.

Then I started to not be able to go the training sessions because I was so tired. Again I was struggling to get out of bed in the mornings and then some days I would just be wide awake and feel like I could do anything.

Then one morning I woke up to play Hockey. All through this I'd never missed a match. It was sunny and was a great day to be playing. I got out of bed fine but I just couldn't go. I still don't know why. I felt like there was just a block to me getting any further than out of bed. I knew something was wrong. I don't know why I did but I just knew.

I went to my GP and she was really helpful. She made me realise that I probably hadn't properly talked to anyone since my mum had been diagnosed. She diagnosed me with depression. She was really positive about it and I started my anti-depressant therapy and started some counselling.

The first week of anti-depressants is hellish. Your emotions are everywhere and your head feels like it's going to explode with all the things that are happening in your every day life. I didn't ring home all that first week. This worried my mum and when I finally told her what had happened she cried. I didn't know how to handle this and I suppose it's only a natural reaction by a mum who thinks that because her child is depressed she's failed them. This is still hard for her to accept but we talk about it a lot and I feel like I can really open up to her now about everything and it's good because she prompts me to open up more to her so we don't get into a situation like before.

Since this first week of taking anti-depressants I've felt much better. The doctor has done some tweaking of my medication and sometimes when this has happened I've felt low for about a week again but on the whole it's really working. I feel more in control. I can concentrate on what I want to do and I can do the things I want to do when I want to do them. Yeh we all have days when we can't get out of bed but I feel like now I have a normal amount of those or they're for a reason such as a late night.

I do all my hobbies and my work without my mood or lack of motivation holding me back.

**

I wrote this because Cancer is still a topic no-one talks about. This book has been hard for me to write and there is a lot of emotion in here that I've struggled to share before now. You're always told that family are around you at your time of need but what happens if this has a massive effect on your family? They need support too and I hope that this shows the importance of having a massive support network.

I also hope that it makes people recognise that emotionally detached isn't right. Teenagers understand what is happening and sometimes feel that they have to be strong like adults when emotionally the experience is affecting them like a child.

If you're reading this as a teenager who's going through the same as me then don't stay in the dark. It's taken me years to come to terms with my experience – don't make the same mistake.

This is part of my healing process. Thanks for reading.

www.ingramcontent.com/pod-product-compliance
Lightning Source LLC
Chambersburg PA
CBHW070255290526
45789CB00004B/1870